Parenting Children
with Health Issues
and Special Needs

Foster W. Cline, MD
& Lisa C. Greene

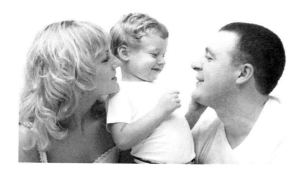

Love and Logic®
Essentials for
Raising Happy,
Healthier Kids

The information published is the opinion of Epic, LLC only and is not meant to supplant or replace professional medical or mental healthcare. Medically-based reasons for behavioral problems should always be considered first.

Original concept design by Pneuma Books LLC; www.pneumabooks.com
Cover, interior design and cartoon illustrations by LisaNortonDesigns.com
Cover photography courtesy of 123RF. Project managed by Lisa C. Greene

Library of Congress Cataloging-in-Publication Data

Cline, Foster.
  Parenting children with health issues and special needs : love and logic essentials for raising happy, healthier kids / by Foster Cline & Lisa C. Greene.
      p. cm.
  ISBN 978-1-935326-04-5
  1. Chronically ill children--Care--Popular works. 2. Children with disabilities--Care--Popular works. I. Greene, Lisa C. II. Title.
  RJ380.C622 2009
  618.92--dc22
                                    2009038648

 Published and printed in the United States of America

"Hope sees the invisible,
feels the intangible, and
achieves the impossible."

- unknown

What are people saying about the unabridged version of "Parenting Children with Health Issues"?

Winner 2008 Indie Excellence Award *(Parenting and Family)*
Winner 2008 Gold Mom's Choice Award *(Health, Nutrition, Fitness, Safety)*
Finalist 2007 ForeWord Magazine's Book of the Year *(Parenting)*

"Shows readers how to help kids identify themselves as having a disease instead of being one." **Library Journal Review**

"An invaluable, experience-laden guide accessible to parents and caretakers of all backgrounds; highly recommended." **Midwest Book Review**

"A highly readable how- to book for parents looking to support the emotional development of their ill children." **Stanford Health Library**

"I literally felt as though you had been sitting in the corner of my exam rooms for all 180,000 office visits. Required reading for families and providers of children with healthcare needs." **Tracy L. Trotter, MD, Fellow of the Amercian Academy of Pediatrics**

"A beacon of insight and guidance for parents in the most challenging of parenting circumstances." **Frazier King, MD, Board Certified Family Practitioner**

"A unique and thorough guide to critical aspects of child-rearing that are just not found anywhere else. It is a gem." *Laura E. Marshak, Author (with Fran Prezant) of: "Married with "Special-Needs Children"*

"Offers a fresh look at the future as well as the possibility of a more joyful day to day life." *Pamela Wilson, BellaOnline's Special Needs Children*

"Radiates with love and good humor; an approach worth studying." *Terri Mauro, "Your Guide to Parenting Special Needs"; About, Inc.*

"For families facing critical health challenges, these practical and proven strategies for effective communication build a foundation for moving on with life." *Carroll Jenkins, Executive Director, Cystic Fibrosis Research Inc, and step-mom of an adult with CF*

"Captures the many thoughts, concerns, challenges and questions I have heard from families living with cystic fibrosis. We need this!" *Beverley Donelson, Co-founder of CF Pharmacy, Inc. and grandmother to a young adult with cystic fibrosis*

"I sure wish this book was available when my children were babies." *Kathy Hardy, mother of eight; three with cystic fibrosis and CF related diabetes*

For additional comments, articles and more, visit:
www.ParentingChildrenWithHealthIssues.com

Introduction

If you are like most parents with a special needs child, you sometimes feel at a loss and don't know what to do. We've been there, too. That's why we wrote our original book *Parenting Children with Health Issues* by Foster Cline, MD and Lisa Greene (Love and Logic Institute, 2007).

We have received numerous letters of appreciation from parents and professionals for the book, and many requests for a more concise version so this is it. Of course this booklet cannot cover everything in *Parenting Children with Health Issues*. However, it will introduce you to the application of Love and Logic® concepts to children with special needs. We believe that it will also inspire you to delve more deeply into the Love and Logic tools and techniques that have proven so effective for parents and teachers over the last three decades.

The term "special needs" encompasses a wide range of physical and developmental issues. When we wrote our book, we focused on children with special healthcare needs like diabetes, cystic fibrosis, allergies, etc. However, we have received much feedback that the concepts have been very helpful to families with special needs of all types, including autism spectrum disorders, developmental delays, mental illness, learning difficulties, etc. That's because our material focuses on family dynamics and parental responses rather than on the specifics of an individual condition.

You'll be discovering communication tools and concepts which are grounded in sound psychology and years of research. Most of the skills work with most children most of the time. However, Love and Logic makes some important assumptions:

- That parents are psychologically healthy
- That parents love their children and want to do what's best for them
- That parents enjoy (or can learn to enjoy) being involved with their children
- That the children are capable of love and causal (if/then) thinking

Even if some of these assumptions are not true, Love and Logic may still be the best and most effective response; however, other measures may be helpful such as psychological counseling, psychotropic medication and behavior modification techniques. These interventions, however, are beyond the scope of this work.

Of course each family is different. We are confident that you'll be able to modify the core concepts to fit your particular situations. Consult with your pediatrician if you are unsure if a tool or technique is appropriate for your child.

Our goal is to provide you with a useful, immediately implementable skill set that will be sufficient for most parenting situations, but will also complement other tools, skills and practices that you may find effective in your own family.

We hope this work will open the door for you to explore the joys of responding effectively to children with special needs. We also invite you to visit **www.ParentingChildrenWithHealthIssues.com** and **www.loveandlogic.com**, where you will find free articles and audio downloads, videos and other resources.

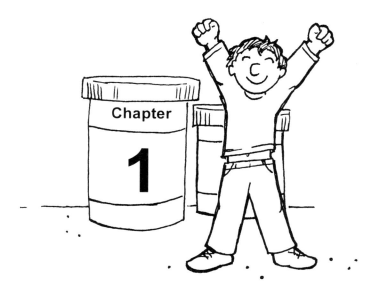

Welcome to Love and Logic!

Congratulations on taking this step to raising children who are confident, respectful, and responsible; children who take responsibility for their own healthcare and fulfill their potential for living fruitful, healthy and happy lives.

This is the "No Guilt" Zone

When parents read a new parenting book or take a class, some might feel regret or guilty when they learn something they wish they had known earlier. That's natural for parents who really care. But relax! Kids are very resilient. The hardest part is often for us parents – getting our old habits out of the way.

Whatever we experienced as children often comes naturally to us when we become parents. As children, many of us were nagged, yelled at, criticized, and punished. So, we either tend to parent our kids in the same way or to do the exact opposite.

It can take a little time and effort to replace those old habits with new ones. Love and Logic makes it easier by offering a model of healthy parenting and the skills to imitate it.

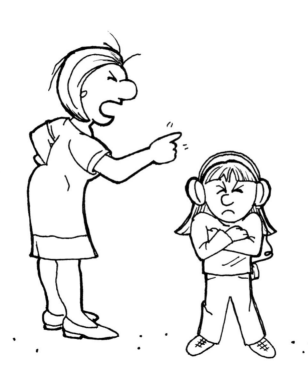

Keep in mind that you are doing the best you can with the information, resources and support you have. We are continually in the process of becoming better parents. That's why you're reading a book on parenting instead of doing something else. And with each new parenting experience, we learn something. So: no guilt.

We are certain that you're doing a lot of things right so feel good about that! Pat yourself on the back every now and then. You deserve it. Parenting can be tough.

Where's the Instruction Manual for this Kid?

Our child is born. We are excited and joyful. Then we get the diagnosis, either before we take the baby home, or a few months or years later. Either way, we find out that our child has a special need or health issue. We grieve. We might feel confused, overwhelmed, depressed or angry. Some of us reach out to loved ones for support, others shut them out. Some devour information about the medical condition and others choose not to.

Our reaction depends on our personality traits, background, and culture. Eventually, most of us reach a point of acceptance. This doesn't mean we are happy with the situation; it just means that we have come to terms with

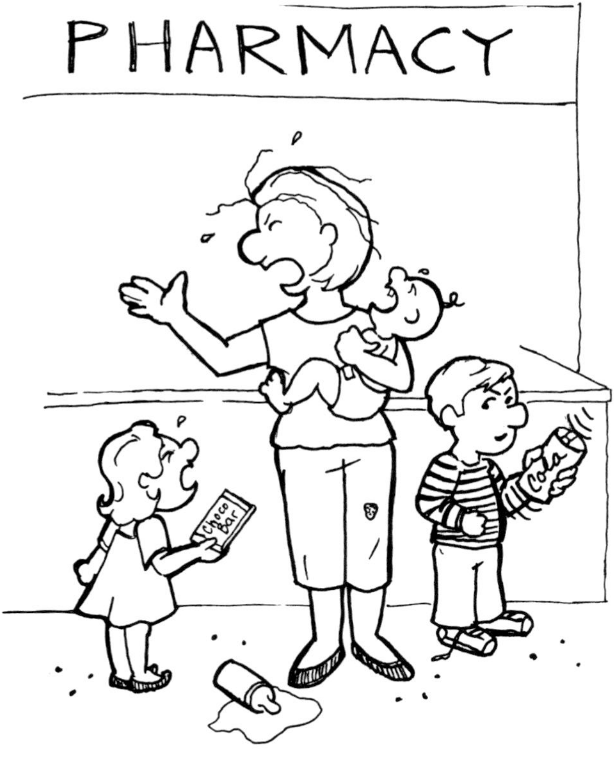
PHARMACY
Choco Bar
Cola

our new reality and have decided to pick ourselves up by our bootstraps and move forward.

This also doesn't mean that we won't sometimes be overwhelmed by our emotions. Life has its ebbs, flows and even some whirlpools that threaten to suck us under. But simply going with the current often gets us to calmer waters. The routines of daily life have a way of taking over.

Depending on your child's age and the severity of condition, you are managing schoolwork, extracurricular, and social activities for your special child and siblings. Plus you have your own responsibilities at home and at work. Then there are doctors' visits, therapists, insurance issues and medications to manage. But, with some organization and cooperation, family life can become enjoyable even with all of the demands that a child's special needs can bring. People and families are amazingly adaptable.

The problem is that it doesn't take much to throw sand into the works and bring it all to a grinding halt: a long-term hospitalization, surgery, or adding another therapy to an already packed schedule. Life can get pretty stressful. With this extra stress comes more frustration!

Isn't it amazing that our kids seem to know when we are the most frazzled and at the end of our rope? And aren't they geniuses at picking that moment to have some "problem"?

Parents can easily feel overwhelmed and wonder, "Where's the instruction manual for this kid? What do I do now?" When a child has special needs, this question is harder to answer without some outside guidance. Love for their special child, coupled with fear, guilt and worry cause parents to act in ways that are more likely to put their child at risk.

It helps to remember the ultimate goal of parenting: *to prepare our kids for the real world.* When we refer to a child "at risk," we mean a child who is not capable of functioning in the real world with all of its choices and consequences.

There are no guarantees that our kids will always make the best decisions. However, by using simple, effective skills, parents can increase the odds of raising confident, responsible kids with excellent coping skills. Wise parents realize that the transition to adulthood begins when their child is old enough to throw peas from the high chair!

Preparing our special children for the real world is the biggest job we will face. That's what Love and Logic is all about: getting our children ready to leave home, to live independently and to know they are not at risk. We want them to look at the real world and say:

"I recognize this world! We practiced for it at home!"

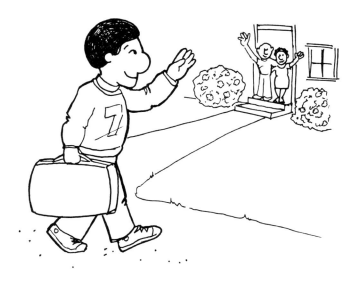

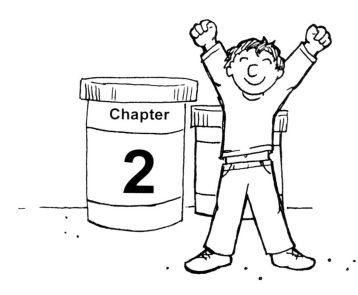

What's the Issue Here?

Do you ever wish you had kids who would eat right, make good decisions, and take responsibility for their healthcare without you having to nag?

Some parents think, "That's impossible" or "I can't believe my child could handle such responsibility." If you do, you might be in for a happy surprise. After reading this booklet, we believe you might even look forward to the next time that your child pushes your buttons because you'll know just what to do. Yes, you will!

Over the years, we've seen this material change the lives of thousands of families, including our own. We can relate to the challenges, and the joys, that you have experienced with your kids. Dr. Cline had a daughter with childhood asthma and another who developed Type I diabetes. Lisa has two children with cystic fibrosis (CF) who between them take about 14 different prescriptions each day, including three that are inhaled. They also do daily chest physical therapy and have special dietary requirements.

At the time of this printing, the median life expectancy for people with CF is thirty-seven but medical advances continue to provide great hope. The odds are good that Lisa's kids will outlive her but their outcome depends on many factors – and especially on how well they take care of themselves.

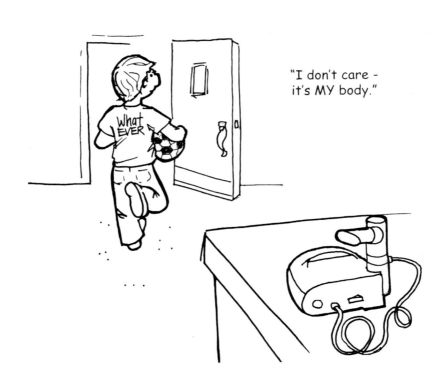

Unfortunately, getting kids to take care of themselves is not easy, particularly when the care is time-consuming or uncomfortable for them.

An all-too-common scene:

"Hey David! Time to do your breathing treatments!"

"Awwww Mom, why?"

"Because if you don't you'll get sick and then you'll have to go to the hospital."

And then he replies, "I don't care- it's my body."

"Well, I'm the one who has to take care of you when you're sick and pay the medical bills! So you need to take care of yourself and you need to ...."

"But I don't wanna. I wanna go out with my friends!"

Sound familiar?

Just once, wouldn't you like to hear, "Thanks for the enlightenment, Mom! My good health is so important to both of us. I'll jump right on it!"

Maybe in our dreams! So the issue comes down to this: how do we get to the point where children do not need reminders, threats or warnings and good self-care including medical adherence becomes *your child's* responsibility, not yours?

Welcome to Love and Logic!

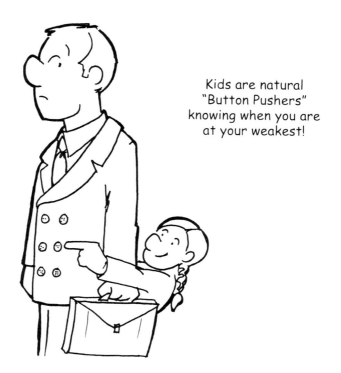

Kids are natural
"Button Pushers"
knowing when you are
at your weakest!

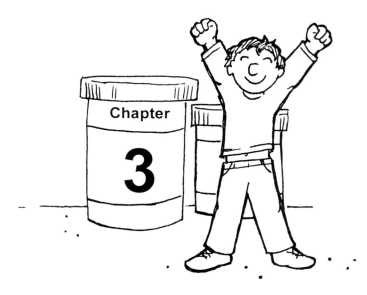

Chapter

3

Avoiding the Bumps in the Road

Parenting isn't for the faint-hearted! Raising kids throughout their developmental stages is tricky enough; parents of kids with special needs have to face additional challenges along the way. When we know where the bumps and potholes are, it becomes a lot easier to avoid them! So let's take a look at some of the challenges parents face when raising kids with medical issues and other special needs.

Who Owns the Problem?

All of Love and Logic's tools and skills are designed to help your children accept responsibility for their own lives including their healthcare. The Love and Logic concept of "who owns the problem" is critical when dealing with chronic illness and the need for good self-care.

The more that parents take ownership of a child's problem, whether it's homework or medication, then the less ownership the child takes. It's like the child unconsciously says, "Well, if Mom or Dad is going to do all of the worrying, I don't need to." And some kids even come right out and say it!

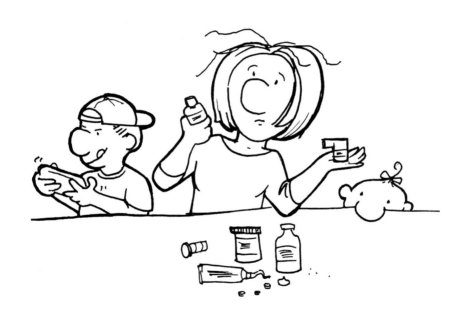

Naturally, when a child is young, or when the condition is life-threatening, a parent *must* take all of the responsibility for the child's care. However, this must change as the child matures. The problem is that most parents don't know when this change should start; the answer is "as early in the child's life as possible."

Of course, we aren't saying that parents should dump all of the responsibility for medical management on the shoulders of a four year old! However, by the time the child is in the 4th or 5th grade, he or she should be expected to remember, at the very least, to take their medications and eat properly. Does this mean 100% of the responsibility? Of course not! But it does mean at least 51%, depending on the maturity and development of the child. So, average 10- or 11-year olds should be well on their way to remembering to take their pancreatic enzymes, test their blood sugar, or check food labels to see if something contains peanuts.

If a parent does not make this transition during the pre-teen years, then as the child enters high school, he or she will be at greater risk of illness or even death due to medical non-compliance or high risk behavior.

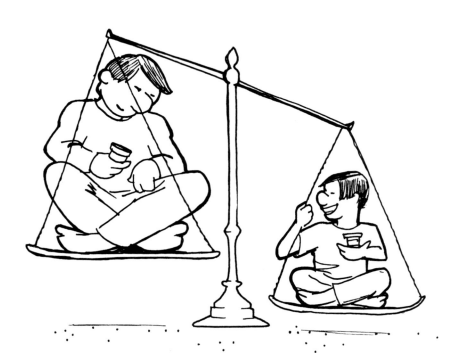

Many parents wait until their child is a teenager before they start turning over the responsibility for self-care to the child; some even wait until their child is heading off to college. Some of these families are successful in these transitions. At the same time, it is all too common to hear stories of children with cystic fibrosis or diabetes who experience a steep deterioration in their health during their first year of college when they are finally out from under their parents' watchful eyes and hands-on involvement.

If children have learned early on that the quality of their lives and health depend upon the choices they make about their self-care, then they will be more likely to make good choices when in a new and exciting environment away from home.

Lisa Greene notes,

> I can't overstate the importance of the concept of the early transferring of responsibility for kids who have a serious chronic disease like CF or diabetes where self-care is critical. And I know it's hard, parents. It can be really hard to let go of something that we think we should be able to control but in reality, really can't.

And I have to say that I have story after story with my own kids where giving up control, sometimes requiring a leap of faith, was absolutely the right thing to do.

It's hard to let go. My children are still fairly young so I want to be careful not to lay too much responsibility at their feet but it is important, even at ages 8 and 10, to have the scale definitely tipped in their direction. And they do a wonderful job of taking responsibility for their care. They pretty much manage their own breathing treatments each day and are working towards managing their other medications, too.

So my point here is that even elementary- aged kids can take responsibility for many aspects of their care and do a good job of it. And, even with all of the helpful tools you're learning, it can be a struggle. Raising kids with health issues just isn't easy. But having effective skills makes a big difference.

Do You Excuse Misbehavior Because of Illness?

Chronic illness and pain can make *all* of us difficult to be around. We can be short-tempered or whiny and that's certainly understandable. At the same time, our sympathy, as parents and caregivers, can lead us to excuse too many behaviors.

Children get very frustrated over the amount of time and energy they spend doing breathing treatments, monitoring blood sugar, or doing physical therapy. Children can easily slide into the "It's not fair" routine and they're right. It's not! And we feel bad for them so we can all to easily over-validate their frustrations.

However, the way that you respond to your children in those moments is what they are going to remember for the rest of their lives. Will they come to see themselves as victims of their medical condition or will they claim victory over it?

Guilt and sympathy, which are always just around the corner, can cloud even the best parenting intuition and judgment. This can cause parents, and everyone else, to tolerate disrespect, misbehavior and poor self-care. Caregivers might even let some of the medical requirements slide, which gives kids the message that it isn't important.

Illness Leads Parents to Feel Frustrated and Everyone Feels a Lack of Control

Control is like food and water: a basic human need. Children who have a chronic medical condition have less control over their time and body. In their frustration, such children can take advantage of their situation and become more demanding.

When children complain or neglect their healthcare, parents naturally become frustrated and may respond by nagging, ranting, raving, rescuing or punishing. This can set up a downward spiral because *when one demands, the other resists!* Who is in control? Parents try to assert control, kids try to regain theirs. The result is a vicious power struggle that the parents rarely win.

When a child is not complying with medical requirements, parents commonly react with frustration and anger. In reality, though, fear is often the underlying emotion. There's a lot to be afraid of when a child has a serious medical condition: fear of the future, fear of declining health, fear of death; the list is endless.

Beneath that fear is another fear: the fear of loss of control. Parents hope that if they can control all medical responsibilities, then things will work out and the kid will stay healthy. What actually happens is that the more parents worry, the less their kids care! "Since Mom and Dad are taking care of that, then I don't need to."

This leads to medical non-adherence and a lack of responsibility. So what do we do? Parents need to make sure their kids take care of themselves, right? We can't just let them not do it. But the key is in the *way* we do it: our parenting style.

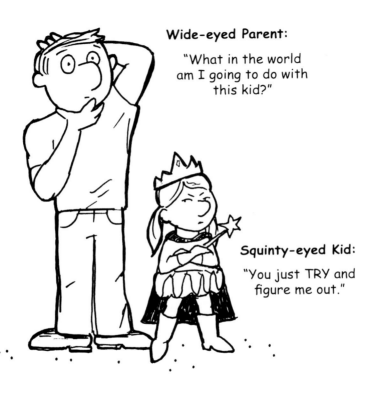

The Development of Healthy Relationships

Parenting style is the way that parents respond to their kids. It can shape the way that kids think and feel about themselves, how hopeful they are about their lives, how resilient they are and how responsible they become. These are all important qualities in children with special needs.

Of course we're born with certain personality traits. You probably noticed that your kid was high energy or perhaps easy-going coming right out of the chute. Still, parents strongly influence the character their children develop and the traits they show. There are *reciprocal* relationships between parent and child:

- Guilty parents raise blaming kids
- Demanding parents raise rebellious kids
- Pleading parents raise whiny kids
- Wide-eyed parents raise squinty-eyed kids

Let's look at parenting styles that generally don't work out so well in the long run. Then we'll talk about what does. Love and Logic emphasizes three parenting styles: Helicopters, Drill Sergeants and Consultants.

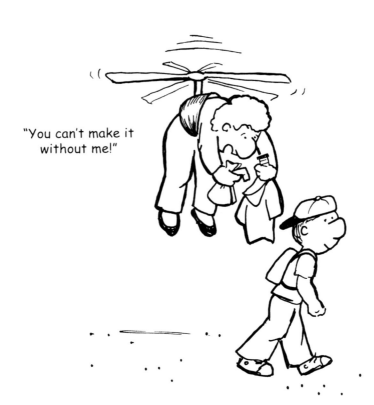

Helicopter Parents

Helicopter Parents hover, rescue and protect.

Parents of children with special needs normally assume hovering and worrying stances. It's unavoidable!

However, the unintended message that helicopter parents can give their children is "You're fragile. You need me to protect you. You can't make it without me!"

These children don't develop confidence in themselves and are much less likely to take responsibility for their behavior and choices. Then the parents take up the slack, the children end up overly dependent and are at a higher risk for depression and/or medical non-compliance.

Helicopter parents blame themselves when things go wrong with their ill children. "What more could I have done?" "Where did I go wrong?" Then, children respond with blame: "It's all *your* fault that I'm so sick. *You* should have done a better job keeping me healthy!"

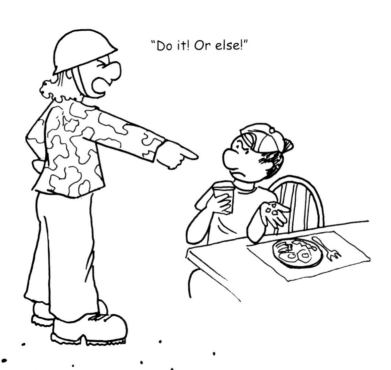

Drill Sergeant Parents

Drill Sergeant Parents use demands and commands.

They say, "Do it! Or else!" Drill Sergeants are necessary on battlefields and in emergency rooms. When kids have problems, Drill Sergeants are right there giving orders and advice.

They take charge out of love but the unspoken message is: "You can't think. I have to do your thinking for you. You aren't capable of making it on your own."

When things go poorly, Drill Sergeant parenting creates resentment. The parent resents the kid for not following orders and the child resents the parent for being bossy.

So Drill Sergeants are in danger of raising angry, rebellious kids who might just choose not to take care of themselves out of spite.

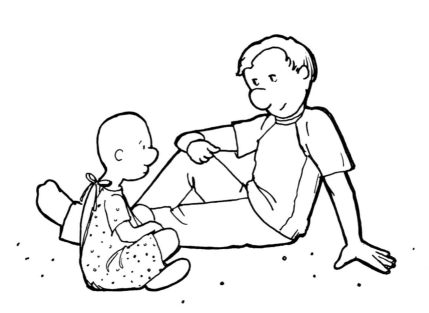

Consultant Parents

*Love and Logic Parents are Consultant Parents. They share their thoughts
and ideas and allow their children to make affordable mistakes.*

Consultants take good care of themselves in front of the children because
they know the importance of modeling. They don't tell kids what to do but
say what *they're* going to do. They offer choices, alternatives, and mutual
problem solving instead of orders and advice. They ask thought-provoking
questions instead of delivering lectures. And they use meaningful actions
laced with empathy instead of nagging, threatening, lecturing, and
rescuing.

Their message is, "You'd best do your own thinking because the quality of
your life has a lot to do with *your* decisions."

Consultant parenting is the only effective style when the use of power is not
an option. Have any of you noticed that teenagers don't deal with "power
trips" well? So, wise parents of adolescents rely on this style-especially
adolescents with health issues.

Our goal is to help you become a Consultant Parent. Read on…

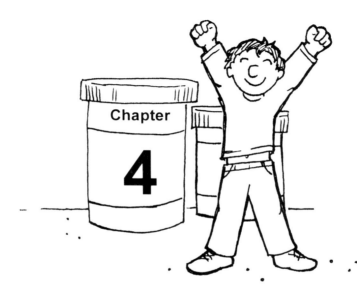

**Whether I think I Can or
Think I Can't, I'm Right!**

Love and Logic tools and techniques build your child's self concept. Self-concept is the way we feel about and see ourselves. This includes perceptions of our personality traits, our skills and abilities, occupations and hobbies, and physical attributes which, for kids with special needs, includes their feelings of victimization, and ability to cope with and meet the challenges of their medical condition or other special need.

Self-concept boils down to two questions: *do we know who we are and do we like what we see?*

It takes a lifetime of effort to "know oneself." Self-concept greatly influences where we will go in life and how we will get there. It determines how we will cope with adversity. It determines whether or not we'll even try something in the first place. Motivation, perseverance, optimism and accomplishment all flow from self-concept.

It is especially important to nurture self-concept in kids that have medical issues. Studies show that people with a high self-concept are more likely to take responsibility for their own healthcare, work harder at medical adherence, have an optimistic outlook, are physically and emotionally healthier, and have more hope. People with low self-concepts tend to give up more easily when they encounter setbacks or obstacles, are more likely to be pessimistic and depressed, and have more health problems.

Of course building a child's self concept is much more complex than this booklet can convey. It is built upon all of the day-to-day interactions and responses over years of living and loving; encouraging and setting high (but reasonable) expectations while being interested and responsive. When parents are Consultants, this philosophy contributes to the development of a child's high self-concept.

What *doesn't* build a high self concept:

- Wealth and material possessions
- Being nice all the time
- Giving children everything they want
- Praising children for a mediocre or poor job
- Not correcting children for misbehavior
- Being a child-centered home where the needs of others are consistently ignored or discounted.
- Rescuing children from their problems

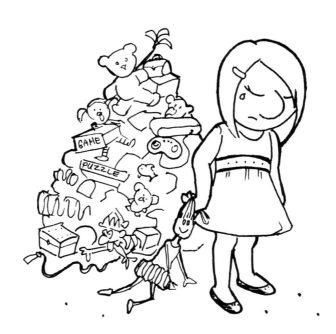

What *does* build a high self-concept:

- Learning to solve problems
- Being able to make choices
- Being treated with respect despite misbehavior
- Helping others and making a difference
- Taking pride in a job well done
- Having effective role models who are "like me"
- Being encouraged and cheered on by others
- Learning how to understand and manage negative emotions

Parents of children with special needs must purposefully nurture their child's self concept. When kids have special needs, they may be limited in physical ability, but must develop unlimited faith in their ability to excel in their areas of strength. Parents might need to be extra creative in engineering situations where their child can be successful. Special Olympics and summer camps are very helpful in this regard. In a safe and nurturing environment, children are developing skills, competing and achieving with others who are living with similar challenges.

What we believe about ourselves defines and creates our reality. Henry Ford said: "Whether you think that you can, or that you can't, you are usually right." Consultant parenting helps raise capable, hopeful kids who *know they can*.

Communicating with Children about Special Needs

Many parents struggle with how and when to give difficult or frightening medical information to their children. Love and Logic principles build character by *assuming that children have the strength and ability to handle the truth when it is given in a loving and caring manner that always allows for hope.*

Wise parents provide accurate information that is appropriate to the child's age and development and empower the child to cope well with what might be difficult news.

Sometimes parents will need to work through their own "stuff" before talking with their child. Children pick up on the parent's attitudes and feelings and take their cues from what their parents say and do. This is especially true of children in the primary grades.

How much information about illness outcomes should parents share with their children? Good answers are honest but are not blunt or insensitive. Children will find out "the truth" one way or another, whether on the internet or from a thoughtless comment by a peer. So, wise parents always tell the truth, answering only the question at hand without volunteering extra information.

So when a *young* child asks, "Will I die from [fill in the blank]?" there is no need to go into the statistics. Simply say something along the lines of: "Well, maybe. But everybody dies of something, and as long as you take good care of your body, you'll most likely live a long and healthy life."

Open parents who are prepared for difficult questions will encourage their children to talk about anything and everything. Such parents radiate an attitude that says "Nothing is too scary for me to talk about. I can handle anything you want to bring to me."

Sometimes it's difficult to talk about tough issues because parents don't know what to say. That's okay! Therapists don't know what they are going to say before they see the client and yet most are very helpful. When you are unsure of how to give the answer, a good technique is to ask more questions.

The following questions can help:

- How much do you know about your illness?
- How worried are you?
- How are you handling it?
- What can I do to make things easier?
- Is there anything more you need to know?
- What special things can you offer others that other kids can't?

Children might not ask certain questions because they want to protect their parents from pain or discomfort. This is why parents need to make sure that children are receiving age- and developmentally appropriate information about their medical condition even if questions aren't immediately forthcoming. It may be helpful to start a discussion with the questions above.

Good communication with ill children always leaves room for hope: "There's a lot of good research being done right now. I know someone with CF who is 72 years old. You take such good care of yourself, you could live a long life, too!"

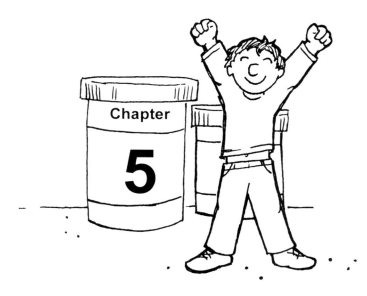

Chapter

5

**Love and Logic Tools for Raising
Healthier Kids**

A foundational belief of Love and Logic is that wise parents offer choices; they do not make demands.

According to human nature, when one demands, the other resists. When we give our kids the right to fail, in areas where the cost is not too high, they are much more likely to choose to succeed. So to avoid, or at least reduce, resistance, parents offer choices and allow kids to make as many decisions as possible; especially when it affects their bodies.

Now of course we're not going to allow a three year old to choose whether or not she will get her flu shot. However, we will let her decide which arm she'd like it in. Older children can decide *when* to do their medical treatments- not *if* they do them.

So parents still set firm limits. Wise adults know which issues to take a stand on and how to set limits in ways that prevent or at least lessen the chance of power struggles. The point is, as much as possible, we make decisions *with* our children, not *for* them.

Choices within limits might be:

- Would you like to do your physical therapy now or after dinner?
- Would you like for us to play a game while you're taking treatments?
- Would you like to have the shot in your right or left arm?
- Honey, do you have a favorite vegetable you'd like for dinner?
- Are you going to do your nebulizer before or after school?
- Would you like to take your medicine with juice or milk?
- Do you plan to have your blood tested tomorrow or Friday?
- Should we have apples or carrots for snack?
- Will you be doing your nasal irrigation right when you get up or after your shower?
- Which would you prefer: lots of butter or half and half in your mashed potatoes?

Choices, choices, choices...

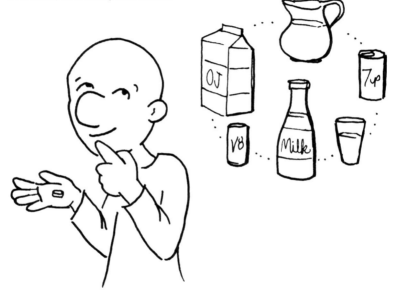

Use lots of little choices like this when things are going well to build up your child's "choice/control savings account." Then, if and when a firm limit must be set, a withdrawal can safely be made: "Don't I usually give you plenty of choices? Yes. Now it's my turn to make one for you. Thanks for understanding."

These are all examples of little choices where the parent is setting the limits and sharing control. As children get older, wise parents use more open ended choices as long as:

- they are confident that the child has good causal thinking (understands that "one thing leads to another").
- the child has the ability to learn from mistakes.
- the consequences of a mistake are not a matter of serious injury or death.

For instance: *parents must make absolutely sure* that children with diabetes take their insulin. However, a child may be given a choice on whether or not to take pancreatic enzymes-a medication which helps digestion. If the child makes an irresponsible choice, he gets a tummy ache and excessive gas. Then the parent can empathetically comment, "Oh, that's a bummer that your tummy hurts. I know it's hard to remember your medication all the time." The child appreciates the empathy and because he or she didn't get "ranting, raving or rescuing" is more likely to remember to take all medication in the future.

When we allow our kids to make decisions about their self care instead of telling them what to do, the responsibility falls onto their shoulders. We empower them to make their own decisions and so they own them as long as we follow through with *empathy and consequences* when they make "bad" choices.

Here's an example from Lisa's family:

> Sharing control with choices is so powerful for developing responsibility. It also helps our relationships to be much more positive! One day, I gave my son the choice to do his breathing treatments in the morning or the evening. He decided to put it off until later in the day.
>
> That evening, a friend called and wanted him to do something special but Jacob couldn't go because he had to get his breathing treatments done. I really wanted to say something like: "I told you so! If only you'd listen to me..." But I was a good Love and Logic

Parent (this time, anyway) and responded with empathy: "Awww, that's a bummer you can't go out with your friend. Maybe it will work out better next time."

It was a tough lesson, but Jake learned at an early age that it's best not to put things off. *He* was responsible for the decision *and* the consequences. Now what would have happened if *I* had decided that he should do the treatments later in the day and he missed out on something fun? He'd be mad at *me* and blame *me*. So allowing *him* to decide avoids blame, resentment and rebellion. *He* makes the mistakes, *he* takes the responsibility.

And in reverse, when he makes the wise decision to get his breathing treatments out of the way early and it works out in his favor, then *he gets the glory*! He feels good about taking care of himself and making wise decisions. So now he is motivated to continue to make good choices.

Every time my kids make a decision, both good and bad, it provides another learning opportunity which will prepare them to be good decision-makers when they're older; when the price tag for mistakes becomes much higher.

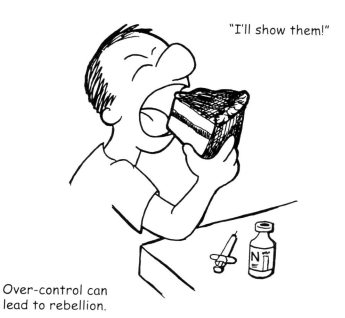

All kids will make mistakes and self-defeating decisions. All of us do, and that's sad. *But it is really sad when children make poor self-care decisions out of rebellion; when they do destructive things to upset a parent.* An example might be skipping their medications or hurting their bodies to get even. Rebellious kids do that. Subconsciously, they think, "You just wait, I'll get even. I'll show you who's *really* boss."

But when parents share the control, allow their kids to make their own decisions as much as possible and respond with empathy rather than anger, then they will greatly reduce the odds that their kids will make self-destructive choices just to get even. When kids "own" their units of concern, they know *they'll* be the one who will ultimately suffer if bad decisions are made.

Using Choices with Food Issues

Food is a big challenge for kids with health issues. In fact, one of the first power struggles for most parents is over getting their toddler to eat. The bottom line is that we can't *make* a kid eat! It drives us crazy when our ill kids won't eat, so it is very easy to get dragged into a power struggle over food.

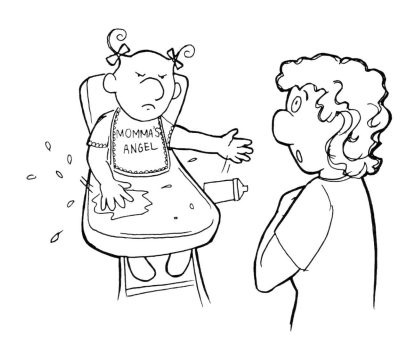

Remember: when one demands, the other resists. So the more you try to *make* your child eat certain foods or a certain amount, the more your child will resist. So, the earlier you start with sharing control of food choices, the better.

Here is a common scenario:

Mom puts the food on the high chair. Toddler Susie takes a bite and says "No. Yucky!" Mom says, "You need to eat." Susie squeezes her lips together . Mom starts to panic so she starts pulling out foods that she knows Susie likes. Anything to get the calories down, right?

"Susie you need to eat. Why won't you eat? Open up! Susie, I said eat!" And on and on. Susie has just been rewarded for being resistant about her food.

Now Susie knows that when she doesn't want to eat, or doesn't like the food, or just wants to make her parents act ridiculous, she just says NO! That leads to treats, attention and *power*. She can even make her dad's face turn red and her mom's voice get really loud! So, it's important not to reward resistance, especially with frustration.

When parents *show* frustration, children's misbehavior is encouraged. This is because showing frustration gives children both emotion and control – the two strongest reinforcements for behavior, good or bad. So the key is to show lots of emotion when your children do things right and very little when they misbehave. Most of us do the opposite. We don't even notice when our kids do things right and then we show all kinds of emotion when they goof up!

So we have to be careful about how we motivate our kids to eat. One way is with choices. Now with younger kids, you can give choices like pancakes or waffles, or one egg or two.

As kids get older, we'll start to give them the freedom to make wider choices. Here's an example from Lisa:

> People with cystic fibrosis need a special diet that is high in calories and fat.
>
> One morning, I asked the kids what they would like for breakfast and they both wanted cold cereal which we don't normally eat for breakfast (we have it around for snacks).

So now *I* had a choice. I could say "No, it's not nutritious enough" and get a fight. Or, I could allow *them* to decide and take this opportunity to teach them by giving them more choices. So, I said, "Okay. You can have cereal but that's only 150 calories and you need 800 for breakfast. Plus, you need some fat, and protein and fruit. So what else will you eat?"

Jacob pipes right up with, "Okay, I'll take peanut butter for my protein and a banana for my fruit. Plus, with a cup of whole milk, that's just about right."

At age ten! And, Kasey decided to have some bacon instead of the peanut butter so everyone was happy.

I realized that if *I* was the one making all the decisions about what they eat and when, then I probably wouldn't be so involved in teaching them. I would just prepare the food and expect them to eat it. *And* end up with a lot of control battles over food. But with choices, I am less likely to have power struggles plus I have a lot more opportunities to teach them along the way.

When my kids are about to make a bad choice, we work through it with questions and more choices so they are empowered to make a better decision. I have found that when we work through it together like this, they rarely make the "bad choice."

If they do, we allow *consequences* to do the teaching rather than lecturing or nagging. Here's an example of the power of choices and consequences:

I was packing my daughter's lunch recently and had put in an oatmeal cream pie which she just loves. She was dawdling over breakfast and I could see that if she didn't hurry it up, she'd run out of time. *I was so tempted to nag!*

Somehow I managed not to. Instead, I simply took the oatmeal pie out of her lunch box and set it on the counter. Then I said, "It looks like you might not finish your breakfast in time so I'm not sure that you'll be able to have this today. I'll set it right here just in case you finish." You should have seen that little mouth move. And she did it! We were both happy and I said, "Way to go, Kasey! You get your yummy cream pie!"

With all of these examples of choices, it might seem that kids get to decide everything. They don't. *Love and Logic Parents are not permissive.* Permissive parents give the kids *all* the control, allowing kids to make choices and decisions even when they irritate or hurt others, including themselves.

Love and Logic Parents allow kids to make many *small* choices. They allow kids to decide things that do not affect or hurt others. The *parents* make the big decisions and the ones that affect the rest of the family. For this, parents need to have some good limit-setting skills.

The most obvious way parents set limits is to say "no" in one form or another. But when we say "no", we get power struggles, whining, arguing, complaining and with some kids, opposition and defiance. So let's learn how to set limits without saying the word "no."

Setting Limits by Using Alternatives to "No"

Say "Yes" Instead...

- Yes! Just as soon as ...
- Absolutely! Right after...
- Of course! And...
- Sure! As long as ...
- Great idea! But first...
- Yes, if...

So say "yes" followed by the limits and conditions you are setting. Here's how it sounds:

"Mom, can I have some cookies?"
"Yes!" [smile and pause] "Just as soon as you finish eating your dinner."

Be sure to put the emphasis on the word "Yes!" It helps to pause and smile. And then say, "as soon as" or "right after" or "but first..."

"YES!"

Here's one for teens: "Hey Mom, can I borrow the car to go over to Bill's house?" "Sure! [pause and smile] Right after you're done with your medical treatments."

This can be a very effective way to set limits and still give our kids hope that they'll get what they want - under the right conditions.

Many of us have kids who are experts at maneuvering us into control battles that there is no way we can win. "Talk to me with respect" is a good example. I mean really, can we *make* our kids talk to us with respect? Or, if they're *really* resistant, can we *make* them take their medications-especially older kids? Not hardly!

So, in our frustration, we often say things to our kids which would be difficult, if not impossible, to enforce. And then when we aren't able to back up what we say, we look like wimps and we lose their respect.

The solution to this is to use **enforceable statements.**

Set Limits with Enforceable Statements

Tell children what *you* are willing to do, not what they have to do:

- I'll be glad to…
- I listen to…
- I'm happy to…
- I drive kids who…
- I will _____ when you _____.

Examples:

Rather than saying, "Don't shout at me," rephrase this to "I'll listen when your voice is soft like mine."

Wrong: Get your treatments done!
Right: I'll be glad to drive you to your friend's house after your medical treatments are done.

Wrong: No drinking and driving.
Right: I'm happy to lend you my car when I don't have to worry about alcohol.

Wrong: Be quiet!
Right: I drive kids to the park as long they are calm and quiet in the car.

Wrong: Eat your food.
Right: I will give you dessert after you finish up your healthy food.

Again, these are all enforceable because we are talking about ourselves and what we will do.

So, in summary, Love and Logic Parents don't set limits with demands, commands and no's. Instead, they use choices, conditional "yesses," enforceable statements and consequences.

How to Neutralize Whining, Arguing and Complaining

Of course no matter how skillful you are at setting limits, some kids will still whine, argue and complain. Love and Logic teaches us two ways to neutralize arguing, whining and complaining.

Option 1: Disarming whines and complaints with empathy

When someone is upset, responding with empathy can be calming. So when a kid says, "Why do I have to check my blood sugar? I hate diabetes," a good response is, "Oh sweetheart, that *is* frustrating. I wish you didn't have diabetes, too. But what might happen if you don't check your blood sugar?" The key is to validate the feelings *and* encourage thinking, wise choices, and correct action. Here are more examples of empathy:

- I'd probably want to do other things than breathing treatments, too, if I were in your shoes.
- It's a bummer at times to have to do things other kids don't have to hassle with.
- I don't blame you for wanting to eat pizza like the other kids.
- That's hard. You sound really frustrated.

Then ask a question that gives your children a choice, but causes them to think and lays the responsibility gently back on their shoulders:

- So how are you going to handle it?
- And what did the doctor say about that?
- Do you worry that if you don't do your medical treatment it could ultimately catch up with you?
- Given your milk allergy, what do you think might happen if you eat that pizza?

Be sure to ask your questions in a loving way with genuine curiosity. Flippant, sarcastic responses will do more harm than good.

Sometimes kids will whine, argue or complain "just because." When they do, it can be very frustrating. Aren't kids *really* good at pushing our buttons? Love and Logic has a solution.

Option 2: Disarming whines and complaints by going brain-dead

A blank stare coupled with a one-liner can put an immediate end to arguing, whining and complaining. The key is not to think about what your child is saying so that you don't get "hooked" into arguing or lecturing. Then, use a one-liner that responds vaguely to disrespectful or negative comments:

- Ummm...
- I bet it feels that way.
- I know.
- Thanks for sharing.
- Probably so.
- Sometimes I'm not sure myself.
- What a bummer.
- Awww. That's sad.
- Well, that's somewhat interesting.
- I love you too much to argue.

One-liners have the advantages that they:

- are irrefutable
- don't tell the child what to do
- are neutral
- can be repeated over and over until the child gives up and wanders off or the adult calmly walks away

They are *not* to be used when a child really wants to engage in a thoughtful conversation or solve a problem. Then, you use the *Steps to Guiding Children to Solve Their Own Problems* shown on page 93.

An example:

Child: "Can I have some popcorn?"

Parent: "Sure! Right after we eat dinner."

Child: "But I want popcorn *now.*"

Parent: "I know and I love you too much to argue."

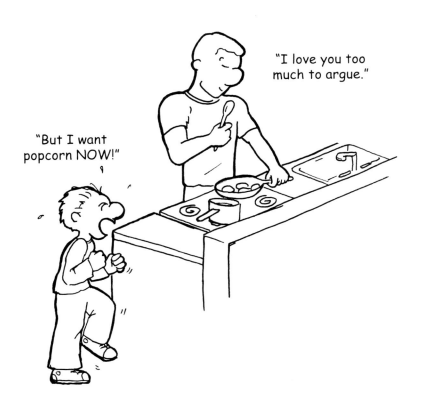

Child: "But I'm *starving.*"

Parent: "Sweetheart, I love you too much to argue."

Child: "Why do you keep saying that?"

Parent: "Because I love you too much to argue!"

(Let's just make sure that we really are concerned about the child's health and the snack really would be unhealthy. Don't use "I love you too much to argue" as a substitute for giving a child's reasonable request reasonable thought.)

And again, avoid the urge to be flippant or sarcastic. They *way* we say things is very important. Tone of voice and body language matter.

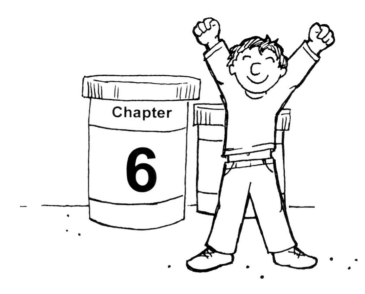

Love and Logic Attitudes

Love and Logic is both a philosophy and a set of practical parenting skills. Skills and attitudes should be mutually supportive. The Love and Logic tools that you have been learning fold into the Love and Logic attitudes. If the attitudes are correct, they almost always lead to naturally using the skills. Conversely, when parents use the skills, they naturally reflect the attitudes of a Consultant Parent.

Love and Logic Attitudes

Sad for, not mad at

Kids make mistakes. Love and Logic Parents see all mistakes as learning opportunities. When a kid misbehaves, wise parents see that as simply another learning opportunity. That is why Love and Logic Parents don't get mad. Instead, they get sad for the child because they know that most mistakes will have some sort of painful experience, or consequence.

Love and Logic Parents respond with *empathy* rather than anger at a child's mistakes and bad decisions. Empathy sounds like, "Oh that's a bummer your stomach hurts. I guess you'll need to stay home from soccer so you can get better." This is very different from "You forgot your enzymes *again*? What did I tell you about taking 'em before you eat? You're grounded!"

Curiosity and interest rather than blame

Rather than being upset at a child's lack of good self-care, Consultant Parents ask *questions* like: "Are you concerned that the way you're treating your body might land you in the hospital?" or "How do you think your liver might be doing right now without its medicine?" Or "Are you thinking you'll be able to do the things you love, like soccer, when you're not taking good care of yourself?"

Questions are very powerful. When we tell children what to do or if we rescue them, we can never really be sure that they are paying attention to us or our message. But when we use questions, it puts the burden for the thinking *on the child*. It also gives us good information about where the training deficiencies might be. Maybe they really *don't* understand why they need to take their medication. So when we ask questions, we can find out what they really know.

Examples of questions that help kids think:

- What could you have done differently?
- How do you think you'll handle it in the future?
- What have you learned from this?
- How do you think you will handle the consequences?

When the parent shows *empathy* toward the child, the result is generally something like: "Gee Mom, thanks for understanding. Next time I'm going to take my pills before I eat."

Empathetic but not excusing

There are many parenting resources out there that emphasize:

- understanding your child
- searching for his or her reasons for misbehavior
- if your children are misbehaving, then understand and nurture them

The importance of giving children love, nurturing, and understanding cannot be over-emphasized. It's absolutely and vitally important. Love is the most important component of all lasting relationships. But giving love and understanding is not the whole story.

In fact, when high functioning and loving parents have trouble with their children, it is generally not because they haven't been loving or nurturing enough. *It is because the parents, in their love, have made understanding the reasons for misbehavior synonymous with excusing misbehavior.*

We'd like to make this point: There are always reasons for misbehavior and reasons for misbehavior can always be understood. In this world, there is much misbehavior by individuals, groups and nations which should be understood… but not excused!

We hear stories from medical professionals about parents who allow their child to be rude, disrespectful and even abusive to medical staff. Just because a child is sick doesn't mean he or she has the right to be nasty– including to parents!

A child not having enough sleep, feeling misunderstood by his teacher, or being chronically ill has plenty of good reasons for treating his mother with a sassy lack of compliance. That doesn't mean she should put up with it or excuse it.

Raising a Victim:
"Eric, I'm going to the store."
"Can I go with you?"
"You were not very nice yesterday in the store."
"Yeah, but I was tired."
"Well, are you going to act that way with me today?"
"No."
"Okay, get your coat."

The child learns: When I'm tired, it's understandable and okay to misbehave. Someday, down the line, it will be "perfectly acceptable" for Eric to scream at his wife if he had a hard day at work.

Raising a Victor:
"Eric, I'm going to the store."
"Can I go with you?"
"You were not very nice yesterday in the store."
"Yeah, but I was tired."

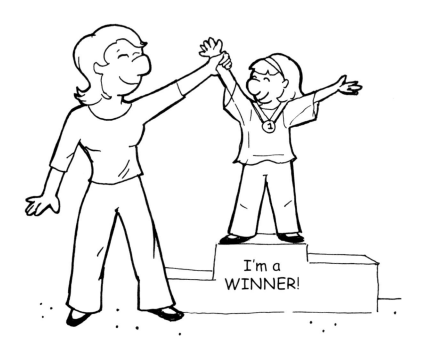

I'm a
WINNER!

"Are you tired today?"

"No."

"Well, that's wonderful! Now your amazing brain can figure out how to get more sleep or control yourself if you are tired. Let me know your thoughts; I'm interested in them. We can chat when I return. See you in a little bit, sweetheart. Bye."

The child learns: "When I am tired my behavior can become unacceptable. Misbehavior has consequences no matter what the reason. I better figure out how to cope with my problems and have self-control.

And *this* child becomes a victor, and hopefully, a leader down the line.

Caring but not rescuing

Let's discuss rescuing. The desire to help others is a wonderful human attribute. Helping others enriches life. Like sugar, helping others adds sweetness to life and may energize us. But too much of a good thing brings an opposite result. Too much sugar leads to diabetes and the possibility of an early death. Too much rescue and help leads to debilitation.

Love and Logic Parents realize that the more problems they solve for their children, the fewer problems their children solve for themselves. Our attitude says, "Honey, I love you, I'm here for you and I'll support you. But I won't rescue you from the problems that you continually cause for yourself."

Love and Logic's **Great Rule for Rescue** is as follows: *It is generally ineffective to go more than half way for a chronic problem people have caused themselves.*

Notice that the **Great Rule** says that it is generally safe to go more than halfway for an acute or chronic problem that people *have not caused themselves.* So when kids are taking responsibility and making good decisions, then of course, help your children in all ways possible.

When life and death are at stake, parents *must always* rescue. We don't let kids go into insulin shock because they weren't monitoring their blood sugar. In such cases, we rescue first and then use imposed consequences to do the teaching.

For example, if a kid refuses to monitor her blood sugar, the parent takes over and does it for her. However, the parent will use *imposed consequences* to do the teaching afterwards: "Feel free to leave the house as long as your blood sugar is being controlled. We can't take the risk of you going into insulin shock while we're not around to help." Or "Honey, I have some bad news for you. You'll be having a chaperone with you everywhere you go until I see that you are managing your blood sugar properly." For a teenager, having a constant adult companion for a few days is a powerful incentive to change!

Dr. Dana Hardin, a leading pediatric endocrinologist, advises parents of resistant kids with diabetes to take them to the doctor or urgent care clinic if they refuse their insulin shots. As Love and Logic teaches, the imposed consequences would be paying a portion of the medical bill.

A great Love and Logic tool is the "Energy Drain" because it gives adults a practical way of modeling good self-care and creating a related consequence for behaviors that might otherwise be hard to find. Just about any misbehavior our kids might do can drain our energy, right?

Let's take a quick look at the steps for the **Energy Drain**:

Step 1: With empathy, inform the child of your energy drain. "Oh Sweetie, this is so sad. When you don't check your glucose levels on time, it drains my energy."

Step 2: Ask the child how he or she will replenish your energy. "How are you planning to put my energy back?"

Step 3: If they don't know, offer them some ideas. "Some kids decide to clean the bathrooms. Other kids decide to mop the kitchen floor. What would you like to do?"

Step 4: Allow them to learn from both success and mistakes.

Some situations are critical but the danger is not imminent such as inhaled antibiotics for a child with CF. In situations like this, before automatically going into rescue mode, Love and Logic Parents first try problem solving.

Steps for Guiding Children to Solve Their Own Problems:

Step 1: Give the child a sincere dose of empathy: "What a bummer to have to stop and do your nebulizer at camp. That must be frustrating."

Step 2: Send the *Power Message*: "But a kid like you can probably handle this with no problem. What do you think you can do?"

Step 3: Offer choices: "Some kids wait until craft time to do them. Other kids wait until after bedtime. And some kids eat dinner real fast and get them done then."

Step 4: Have the child state the consequences for each choice: "How would that work for you?"

Step 5: Lovingly give permission for the child to solve or not solve the problem. "Gosh, you could handle it this way or that, or I guess you could do nothing. But that might not work out well for you. Let me know what you decide to do; good luck."

Love and Logic Parents allow the child to learn from his or her mistakes as long as there is no immediate danger. If a child makes a bad decision (like doing nothing), then imposed consequences will do the teaching such as, in the above example, having the child do the breathing treatments at an inconvenient time like late at night or during a favorite activity or, as a last resort, leaving camp early.

Show acceptance without necessarily showing approval

All people yearn for acceptance. When parents are able to show acceptance without necessarily indicating approval, children appreciate their parents as a wise counselor – someone to go to when times are tough or when mistakes have been made rather than someone to hide from.

Examples:

Parents control their body language and make sure that they are open and curious and say things like:

- Gosh sweetheart, I hope that works out okay.
- Hmmm, well, I would have done it differently.

- I understand you are happy about your decision, but I'm having a hard time understanding that.
- Let me know how that works out for you. I'm a little concerned about it.

Each one of these phrases implies: "I don't agree with you but I am accepting the fact that it's your life and you need to decide how to handle it." When this is coupled with empathy and allowing the children to work through the consequences of their decisions, parents encourage love and respect.

If your child makes a bad decision and things go wrong, avoid saying, "I told you so. You should have listened to me." Instead, be empathetic: "Aww, that's a bummer it didn't work out like you expected it to. Now what?"

• • •

Now you see how Love and Logic attitudes blend with Love and Logic tools and techniques. They all complement each other and flow together to create consistency in parenting responses and discipline.

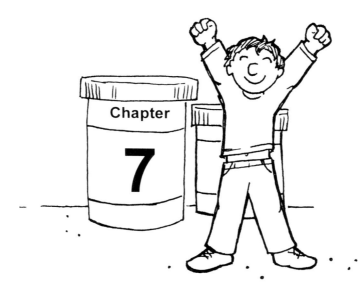

The Power of Love

This booklet wouldn't be complete if we didn't mention two core aspects of parenting kids with special needs: caregiver self-care and the importance of relationships. We cover both issues thoroughly in our book *Parenting Children with Health Issues* so we won't go into much detail here. Suffice it to say that, as caregivers, we sometimes get so busy focusing on the needs of everyone else, that we put ourselves last. This can be dangerous.

Burnout and depression among caregivers is common. When the primary caregiver is burned out, medical adherence and quality of life for the entire family suffers. As we've discussed, kids pick up their cues from parents, so we encourage you to take good care of yourself and consider your own needs to be just as important as everyone else's.

Along those lines, we can get so busy with managing the details of our child's special needs, plus everything else that life throws at us, that we forget to nurture our relationships with our children and significant other.

Dr. Charles Fay of Love and Logic says, "Rules without relationship lead to rebellion. Consequences without relationship lead to resentment. Rewards without relationship feel like bribes. It's the *relationship* we have with our kids that makes consequences and limits work. When our kids are bonded to us, that's what makes the difference."

Make showing your love a priority. Spend time playing with your kids and having fun. Notice what they do right more than what they do wrong. Tell them you love them. Listen to their stories, hopes and dreams. Smile at them and laugh with them. Childhood is magical...

Never underestimate the power of love to heal and bring hope.

When Helen Keller became deaf and blind at nineteen months of age due to illness, she became like a wild animal. Many people gave up on her and told her mother to put her into an institution because there was no hope.

Her mother refused to give up. The story of how a teacher named Anne Sullivan brought light to Helen's world of darkness has inspired generations. So don't give up! Keep on loving and keep on hoping.

Because: "Hope sees the invisible, feels the intangible, and achieves the impossible."

Our thoughts and prayers go with you on your parenting journey. We know that you, like us, will face challenges. We hope that, despite the trials, you find peace, joy and many blessings as you raise your special child to be all that he or she can be.

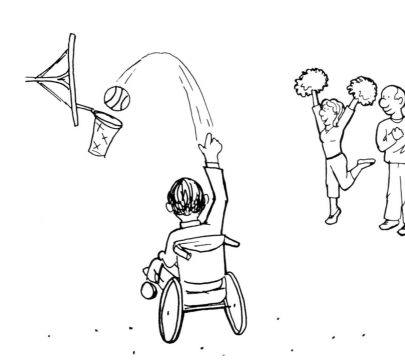

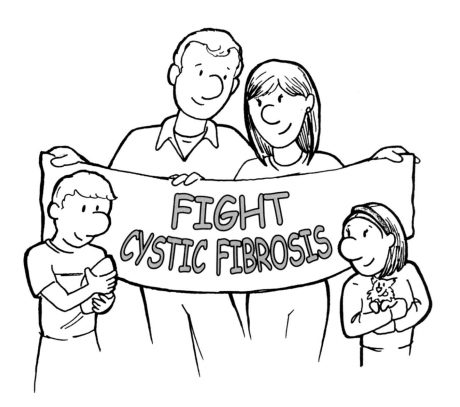

Thank you!

Thank you to the many parents and children who have shared, helped, and inspired us over the years as we have worked on this important program. We are also grateful to the many medical and mental health professionals who have given us their ideas and feedback and have helped spread the word about us. Most of all, we are grateful to our families for helping us with the details of bringing a new book into the world and sharing in the joys and struggles of life.

We especially thank Jacob and Kasey Greene who have graciously given us their permission to share their stories with you. They continue to inspire and teach us.

Last, but never least, we are very grateful for the hope that the possibility of a cure for CF brings. For this, we thank the Cystic Fibrosis Foundation, Cystic Fibrosis Research Inc, The Boomer Esiason Foundation and the thousands of professionals around the world that work tirelessly to take good care of us and find the cure.

Co-author Lisa Greene will donate her share of the proceeds from this booklet to help in the fight for a cure for cystic fibrosis.

Love and Logic Resources

Change takes time and effort. It's best to master one skill at a time. Start with challenges over chores or homework before tackling tougher medical issues. As you try out these new skills and see how well they work, you'll be encouraged to continue working on them. At the same time, it's normal to fall back into old patterns. So take advantage of our resources, many of them free, to stay motivated and keep moving forward.

Order all resources at www.loveandlogic.com or 800-338-4065

General parenting resources by Foster Cline, MD:

Parenting with Love and Logic by Foster Cline, MD and Jim Fay
Parenting Teens with Love and Logic by Foster Cline, MD and Jim Fay
Grandparenting with Love and Logic by Jim Fay and Foster Cline, MD
Marriage Love and Logic by Foster Cline, MD and Hermie Drill Cline

Sign up for the Love and Logic Insider's Club for tips and discounts
Free humorous audio downloads
Podcasts of *The Love and Logic Show*

www.loveandlogic.com

This booklet is a highly condensed version of the book *Parenting Children with Health Issues* by Foster Cline, MD and Lisa Greene.

What can you discover in the original?
- Special Issues for Ages and Stages of Development
- How do Kids Really Learn? The Five E's
- Is it "I Can't" or "I Won't"?
- Relationships: Siblings, Marriage and Family
- Love and Logic Quick Tips Cards
- Inspiring Stories and Lots More….

Other Resources for Parenting Children with Health Issues and Special Needs:

Parenting Children with Health Issues by Foster Cline, MD and Lisa Greene
CD: *Winning with Diabetes* by Foster Cline, MD and Charles Fay, PhD
CD: *Grief, Trauma and Loss: Helping Children Cope* by Foster Cline, MD
DVD: *Parenting Children with Health Issues and Special Needs* DVD Series

Free audio downloads, slide shows and video clips
Free articles, tips, and *Ask Dr. Cline*
Information about workshops and teleclasses

www.ParentingChildrenWithHealthIssues.com

About the Authors

About Foster W. Cline, MD

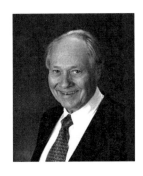

Dr. Cline is the co-founder of the Love and
Logic Institute with Jim Fay. A gifted child
psychiatrist, physician, international speaker,
and author of many books on parenting and
dealing with difficult children and their families,
Dr. Cline has worked with parents and children
for over forty years.

About Lisa C. Greene, BS CCP

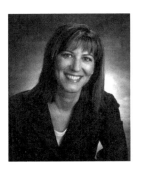

Lisa is the mother of two children with cystic
fibrosis, a certified parent coach, and a parent
educator. She combines her training with
personal experiences and insights and shares
this with you as she raises her two special
children with Love and Logic's essential and
life-changing parenting tools.